VEGETARIAN HIGH PROTEIN RECIPES FOR TYPE 2 DIABETICS

A Plant-Based Protein Guide for Type 2 Diabetes

T. John

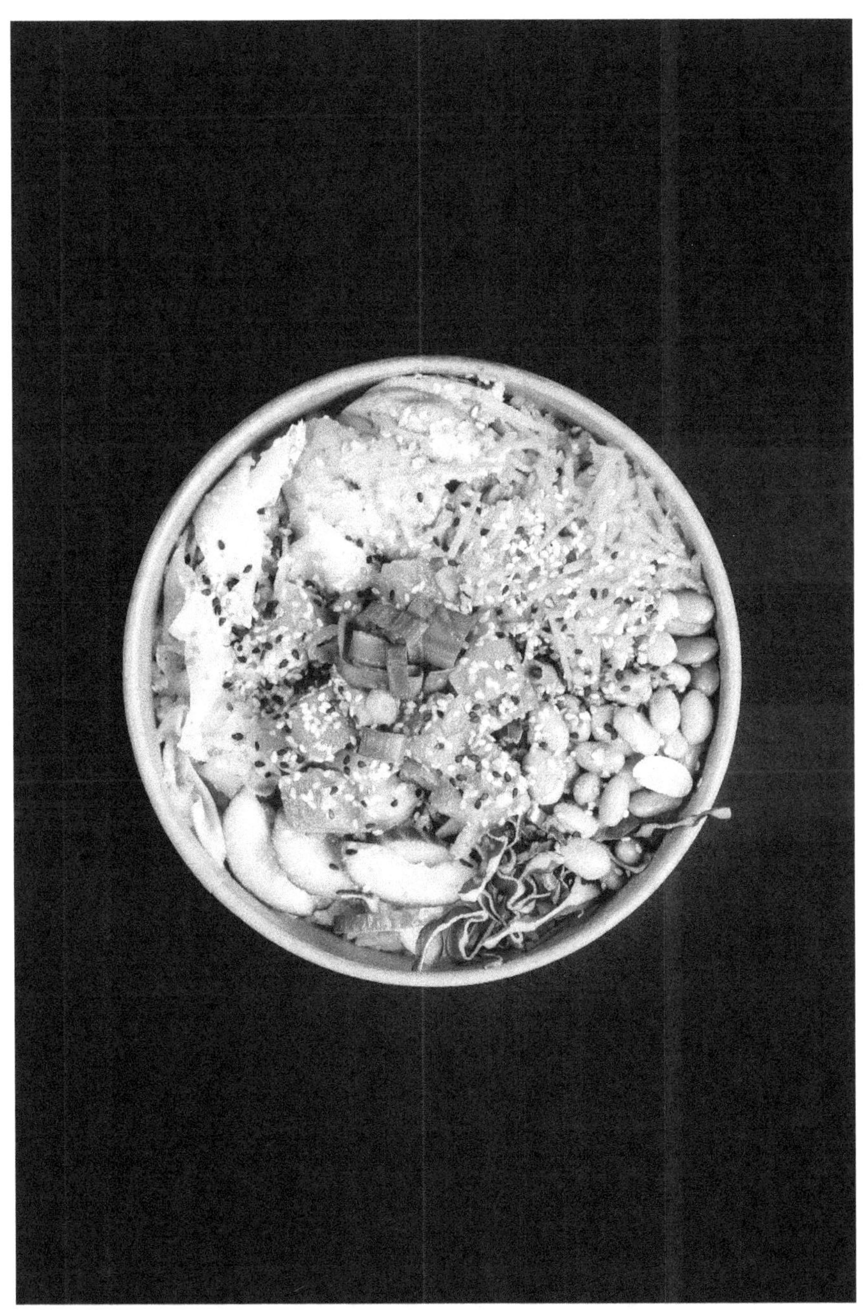

TABLE OF CONTENTS

Chapter 5: Snacks and Appetizers 77

INTRODUCTION

Type 2 diabetes disrupts your body's ability to regulate blood sugar levels. This can lead to a cascade of health concerns. While medication plays a crucial role, dietary choices are a powerful tool in managing the condition. A well-balanced diet focused on whole foods, portion control, and regular mealtimes is key.

The Potential of a High-Protein Vegetarian Diet

For people with type 2 diabetes, a high-protein vegetarian diet can be a game-changer. Here's why:

- **Slower Glucose Release:** Plant-based protein sources like beans, lentils, and tofu are digested at a slower rate compared to animal protein. This translates to a steadier rise in blood sugar levels, minimizing spikes and crashes.

- **Fiber Powerhouse:** Vegetarian meals are naturally rich in fiber, which helps regulate digestion and keeps you feeling fuller for longer. This can be particularly beneficial for managing cravings and maintaining a healthy weight, which further aids blood sugar control.

- **Heart-Healthy Benefits:** Many plant-based proteins are lower in saturated fat than their meat counterparts. This translates to a reduced risk of heart disease, a common concern for diabetics.

Building Your High-Protein Vegetarian Plate

Now, let's explore the building blocks of your delicious and diabetic-friendly meals:

- **Protein Powerhouses:** Beans, lentils, chickpeas, tempeh, tofu, seitan, nuts, and nut butters are your all-stars. Rotate these throughout the week to ensure a variety of nutrients.
- **Fiber Fantastic Vegetables:** Load up on non-starchy vegetables like broccoli, spinach, kale, peppers, and mushrooms. These provide essential vitamins and minerals while keeping your blood sugar in check.
- **Whole Grain Wonders:** Brown rice, quinoa, whole-wheat bread, and barley add sustained energy and essential fiber. Opt for whole grains over refined options whenever possible.

- **Healthy Fat Friends:** Don't be afraid of healthy fats! Include avocados, olives, and nuts for satiety and essential fatty acids.

Substitutions and Creativity in the Kitchen

Worried about missing out on familiar flavors? Here are some creative substitutions:

- **Craving Burgers?** Make veggie burgers with black beans, lentils, or quinoa. Top them with a tangy yogurt sauce for a satisfying twist.
- Missing Meat in Stir-fries? Tempeh or tofu, cubed and marinated, can replace meat while adding a protein punch.
- **Yearning for Eggs?** A chickpea flour omelet, seasoned with turmeric or nutritional yeast, offers a surprisingly eggy flavor and texture.

Planning and Prep: Keys to Success

Meal planning and prepping are essential for a successful high-protein vegetarian diet. Here are some tips:

- **Plan Your Week:** Dedicate time each week to plan your meals and create a grocery list.

- **Prep in Advance:** Cook a large batch of quinoa or brown rice on Sundays. Chop vegetables and store them in containers for easy access during the week.

- **Embrace Leftovers:** Leftovers can be your best friend! Repurpose them into creative lunches or quick dinners.

- **Snacks Matter:** Plan healthy snacks like nuts, seeds, or veggie sticks with hummus to keep your energy levels stable.

Remember: With a little planning and creativity, a high-protein vegetarian diet can be a delicious and empowering way to manage your type 2 diabetes.

Chapter 1: 30 Day Meal Plan

Week 1

Day 1

- Breakfast: Greek Yogurt Parfait with Berries and Nuts
- Lunch: Chickpea Salad with Lemon Tahini Dressing
- Dinner: Black Bean and Quinoa Tacos
- Snack: Roasted Chickpeas
- Dessert: Chia Seed Pudding with Cocoa

Day 2

- Breakfast: Quinoa and Vegetable Breakfast Bowl
- Lunch: Grilled Portobello Mushroom Burger
- Dinner: Eggplant Parmesan with Tofu
- Snack: Edamame Hummus with Veggies
- Dessert: Almond Flour Brownies

Day 3

- Breakfast: Spinach and Feta Omelette
- Lunch: Lentil and Sweet Potato Stew
- Dinner: Chickpea and Spinach Stew
- Snack: Greek Yogurt with Cucumber and Dill
- Dessert: Vegan Protein Cookies

Day 4

- Breakfast: Chia Seed Pudding with Almond Milk
- Lunch: Quinoa and Black Bean Salad
- Dinner: Cauliflower Steaks with Lentil Sauce
- Snack: Spicy Tofu Bites
- Dessert: Greek Yogurt with Honey and Walnuts

Day 5

- Breakfast: Avocado Toast with Chickpeas
- Lunch: Tofu and Vegetable Stir-Fry
- Dinner: Vegan Shepherd's Pie with Lentils
- Snack: Almond and Seed Crackers
- Dessert: Black Bean Brownies

Day 6

- Breakfast: Tofu Scramble with Vegetables
- Lunch: Spinach and Chickpea Curry
- Dinner: Stuffed Acorn Squash with Quinoa
- Snack: Lentil and Vegetable Samosas
- Dessert: Tofu Chocolate Mousse

Day 7

- Breakfast: Cottage Cheese and Fruit Salad
- Lunch: Zucchini Noodles with Pesto and Edamame

- Dinner: Tempeh and Vegetable Kebabs
- Snack: Stuffed Mini Peppers with Quinoa
- Dessert: Peanut Butter Protein Balls

Week 2

Day 8

- Breakfast: Protein-Packed Smoothie Bowl
- Lunch: Roasted Vegetable and Hummus Wrap
- Dinner: Spaghetti Squash with Tomato and Basil
- Snack: Baked Zucchini Chips
- Dessert: Avocado Chocolate Pudding

Day 9

- Breakfast: Oatmeal with Almond Butter and Flaxseeds
- Lunch: Cauliflower Rice and Bean Bowl
- Dinner: Mushroom Stroganoff with Tofu
- Snack: Guacamole with Veggie Sticks
- Dessert: Baked Apple with Cinnamon and Nuts

Day 10

- Breakfast: Vegan Protein Pancakes
- Lunch: Broccoli and Tempeh Salad
- Dinner: Lentil and Mushroom Bolognese

- Snack: Cottage Cheese and Herb Dip
- Dessert: Vegan Protein Cheesecake

Day 11

- Breakfast: Lentil and Vegetable Breakfast Muffins
- Lunch: Stuffed Bell Peppers with Quinoa and Beans
- Dinner: Vegan Moussaka with Eggplant and Lentils
- Snack: Spicy Black Bean Dip with Whole Grain Chips
- Dessert: Chocolate-Covered Almonds

Day 12

- Breakfast: High-Protein Granola with Yogurt
- Lunch: Mushroom and Barley Soup
- Dinner: Butternut Squash and Chickpea Curry
- Snack: Kale and Chickpea Chips
- Dessert: Coconut and Almond Macaroons

Day 13

- Breakfast: Edamame and Veggie Breakfast Wrap
- Lunch: Veggie Sushi Rolls with Tofu
- Dinner: Vegan Pad Thai with Tofu
- Snack: Veggie and Tofu Skewers
- Dessert: Protein-Packed Banana Bread

Day 14

- Breakfast: Baked Eggplant and Tomato Frittata
- Lunch: Mediterranean Lentil Soup
- Dinner: Sweet Potato and Black Bean Enchiladas
- Snack: Almond Butter and Banana Bites
- Dessert: Carrot Cake Bites

Week 3

Day 15

- Breakfast: Almond Flour Breakfast Cookies
- Lunch: Vegan Caesar Salad with Crispy Chickpeas
- Dinner: Cauliflower and Chickpea Tikka Masala
- Snack: Protein-Packed Energy Balls
- Dessert: High-Protein Berry Crumble

Day 16

- Breakfast: Greek Yogurt Parfait with Berries and Nuts
- Lunch: Chickpea Salad with Lemon Tahini Dressing
- Dinner: Black Bean and Quinoa Tacos
- Snack: Roasted Chickpeas
- Dessert: Chia Seed Pudding with Cocoa

Day 17

- Breakfast: Quinoa and Vegetable Breakfast Bowl
- Lunch: Grilled Portobello Mushroom Burger
- Dinner: Eggplant Parmesan with Tofu
- Snack: Edamame Hummus with Veggies
- Dessert: Almond Flour Brownies

Day 18

- Breakfast: Spinach and Feta Omelette
- Lunch: Lentil and Sweet Potato Stew
- Dinner: Chickpea and Spinach Stew
- Snack: Greek Yogurt with Cucumber and Dill
- Dessert: Vegan Protein Cookies

Day 19

- Breakfast: Chia Seed Pudding with Almond Milk
- Lunch: Quinoa and Black Bean Salad
- Dinner: Cauliflower Steaks with Lentil Sauce
- Snack: Spicy Tofu Bites
- Dessert: Greek Yogurt with Honey and Walnuts

Day 20

- Breakfast: Avocado Toast with Chickpeas
- Lunch: Tofu and Vegetable Stir-Fry

- Dinner: Vegan Shepherd's Pie with Lentils

- Snack: Almond and Seed Crackers

- Dessert: Black Bean Brownies

Day 21

- Breakfast: Tofu Scramble with Vegetables

- Lunch: Spinach and Chickpea Curry

- Dinner: Stuffed Acorn Squash with Quinoa

- Snack: Lentil and Vegetable Samosas

- Dessert: Tofu Chocolate Mousse

Week 4

Day 22

- Breakfast: Cottage Cheese and Fruit Salad

- Lunch: Zucchini Noodles with Pesto and Edamame

- Dinner: Tempeh and Vegetable Kebabs

- Snack: Stuffed Mini Peppers with Quinoa

- Dessert: Peanut Butter Protein Balls

Day 23

- Breakfast: Protein-Packed Smoothie Bowl

- Lunch: Roasted Vegetable and Hummus Wrap

- Dinner: Spaghetti Squash with Tomato and Basil

- Snack: Baked Zucchini Chips
- Dessert: Avocado Chocolate Pudding

Day 24

- Breakfast: Oatmeal with Almond Butter and Flaxseeds
- Lunch: Cauliflower Rice and Bean Bowl
- Dinner: Mushroom Stroganoff with Tofu
- Snack: Guacamole with Veggie Sticks
- Dessert: Baked Apple with Cinnamon and Nuts

Day 25

- Breakfast: Vegan Protein Pancakes
- Lunch: Broccoli and Tempeh Salad
- Dinner: Lentil and Mushroom Bolognese
- Snack: Cottage Cheese and Herb Dip
- Dessert: Vegan Protein Cheesecake

Day 26

- Breakfast: Lentil and Vegetable Breakfast Muffins
- Lunch: Stuffed Bell Peppers with Quinoa and Beans
- Dinner: Vegan Moussaka with Eggplant and Lentils
- Snack: Spicy Black Bean Dip with Whole Grain Chips
- Dessert: Chocolate-Covered Almonds

Day 27

- Breakfast: High-Protein Granola with Yogurt
- Lunch: Mushroom and Barley Soup
- Dinner: Butternut Squash and Chickpea Curry
- Snack: Kale and Chickpea Chips
- Dessert: Coconut and Almond Macaroons

Day 28

- Breakfast: Edamame and Veggie Breakfast Wrap
- Lunch: Veggie Sushi Rolls with Tofu
- Dinner: Vegan Pad Thai with Tofu
- Snack: Veggie and Tofu Skewers
- Dessert: Protein-Packed Banana Bread

Day 29

- Breakfast: Baked Eggplant and Tomato Frittata
- Lunch: Mediterranean Lentil Soup
- Dinner: Sweet Potato and Black Bean Enchiladas
- Snack: Almond Butter and Banana Bites
- Dessert: Carrot Cake Bites

Day 30

- Breakfast: Almond Flour Breakfast Cookies
- Lunch: Vegan Caesar Salad with Crispy Chickpeas

- Dinner: Cauliflower and Chickpea Tikka Masala

- Snack: Protein-Packed Energy Balls

- Dessert: High-Protein Berry Crumble

Chapter 2: Breakfast Recipes

A well-balanced breakfast sets the tone for the day, particularly for those managing Type 2 diabetes. These high-protein vegetarian breakfast recipes are designed to keep you full and satisfied while maintaining stable blood sugar levels. Each recipe is crafted to be nutrient-dense, delicious, and easy to prepare.

Greek Yogurt Parfait with Berries and Nuts

Ingredients:

- 1 cup Greek yogurt
- 1/2 cup mixed berries (strawberries, blueberries, raspberries)
- 2 tablespoons mixed nuts (almonds, walnuts, pistachios)
- 1 teaspoon honey (optional)

Instructions:

1. Layer Greek yogurt in a glass or bowl.
2. Top with mixed berries and nuts.
3. Drizzle with honey, if desired.

Nutrition Information:

- Calories: 250

- Protein: 15g
- Carbohydrates: 20g
- Fat: 10g
- Fiber: 4g
- Sugar: 12g
- Portion Size: 1 serving

Quinoa and Vegetable Breakfast Bowl

Ingredients:

- 1/2 cup cooked quinoa
- 1/4 cup diced bell peppers
- 1/4 cup chopped spinach
- 1/4 cup cherry tomatoes, halved
- 1 tablespoon olive oil
- Salt and pepper to taste

Instructions:

1. In a bowl, mix cooked quinoa, bell peppers, spinach, and cherry tomatoes.
2. Drizzle with olive oil and season with salt and pepper.

Nutrition Information:

- Calories: 200

- Protein: 6g

- Carbohydrates: 30g

- Fat: 8g

- Fiber: 4g

- Sugar: 3g

- Portion Size: 1 serving

Spinach and Feta Omelette

Ingredients:

- 2 eggs

- 1/4 cup chopped spinach

- 2 tablespoons crumbled feta cheese

- Salt and pepper to taste

- 1 teaspoon olive oil

Instructions:

1. Beat eggs and season with salt and pepper.

2. In a pan, heat olive oil and sauté spinach until wilted.

3. Add eggs and cook until almost set, then sprinkle feta on top.

4. Fold omelette and cook for another minute.

Nutrition Information:

- Calories: 220

- Protein: 14g

- Carbohydrates: 2g

- Fat: 18g

- Fiber: 1g

- Sugar: 1g

- Portion Size: 1 omelette

Chia Seed Pudding with Almond Milk

Ingredients:

- 1/4 cup chia seeds

- 1 cup almond milk

- 1 teaspoon vanilla extract

- 1 tablespoon maple syrup (optional)

- Fresh fruit for topping

Instructions:

1. Mix chia seeds, almond milk, vanilla extract, and maple syrup in a bowl.

2. Refrigerate for at least 2 hours or overnight.

3. Top with fresh fruit before serving.

Nutrition Information:

- Calories: 180

- Protein: 6g

- Carbohydrates: 18g

- Fat: 9g

- Fiber: 10g

- Sugar: 5g

- Portion Size: 1 serving

Avocado Toast with Chickpeas

Ingredients:

- 1 slice whole grain bread

- 1/2 avocado, mashed

- 1/4 cup canned chickpeas, rinsed and mashed

- Salt, pepper, and red pepper flakes to taste

Instructions:

1. Toast the bread slice.

2. Spread mashed avocado on toast, then top with mashed chickpeas.

3. Season with salt, pepper, and red pepper flakes.

Nutrition Information:

- Calories: 250

- Protein: 8g

- Carbohydrates: 32g
- Fat: 12g
- Fiber: 10g
- Sugar: 2g
- Portion Size: 1 slice

Tofu Scramble with Vegetables

Ingredients:

- 1/2 block firm tofu, crumbled
- 1/4 cup diced bell peppers
- 1/4 cup chopped spinach
- 1/4 cup diced tomatoes
- 1 teaspoon turmeric
- Salt and pepper to taste
- 1 tablespoon olive oil

Instructions:

1. Heat olive oil in a pan and sauté bell peppers, spinach, and tomatoes.
2. Add crumbled tofu, turmeric, salt, and pepper.
3. Cook until tofu is heated through and vegetables are tender.

Nutrition Information:

- Calories: 200
- Protein: 14g
- Carbohydrates: 8g
- Fat: 12g
- Fiber: 3g
- Sugar: 3g
- Portion Size: 1 serving

Cottage Cheese and Fruit Salad

Ingredients:

- 1 cup cottage cheese
- 1/2 cup diced fresh fruit (pineapple, berries, melon)
- 1 tablespoon chopped nuts (optional)

Instructions:

1. Combine cottage cheese and diced fresh fruit in a bowl.
2. Top with chopped nuts, if desired.

Nutrition Information:

- Calories: 200
- Protein: 14g
- Carbohydrates: 18g

- Fat: 8g
- Fiber: 2g
- Sugar: 12g
- Portion Size: 1 serving

Protein-Packed Smoothie Bowl

Ingredients:

- 1 banana, frozen
- 1/2 cup Greek yogurt
- 1/2 cup mixed berries
- 1 tablespoon chia seeds
- 1 scoop protein powder
- Toppings: granola, fresh fruit, nuts

Instructions:

1. Blend frozen banana, Greek yogurt, mixed berries, chia seeds, and protein powder until smooth.
2. Pour into a bowl and add desired toppings.

Nutrition Information:

- Calories: 300
- Protein: 20g
- Carbohydrates: 45g

- Fat: 8g
- Fiber: 8g
- Sugar: 25g
- Portion Size: 1 bowl

Oatmeal with Almond Butter and Flaxseeds

Ingredients:

- 1/2 cup rolled oats
- 1 cup water or almond milk
- 1 tablespoon almond butter
- 1 tablespoon ground flaxseeds
- 1/4 teaspoon cinnamon
- Fresh fruit for topping (optional)

Instructions:

1. Cook oats in water or almond milk according to package instructions.
2. Stir in almond butter, flaxseeds, and cinnamon.
3. Top with fresh fruit, if desired.

Nutrition Information:

- Calories: 250

- Protein: 8g

- Carbohydrates: 35g

- Fat: 10g

- Fiber: 8g

- Sugar: 5g

- Portion Size: 1 serving

Vegan Protein Pancakes

Ingredients:

- 1 cup whole wheat flour

- 1 scoop vegan protein powder

- 1 tablespoon ground flaxseeds

- 1 teaspoon baking powder

- 1 cup almond milk

- 1 tablespoon maple syrup

- 1 teaspoon vanilla extract

- Coconut oil for cooking

Instructions:

1. Mix flour, protein powder, ground flaxseeds, and baking powder in a bowl.

2. Add almond milk, maple syrup, and vanilla extract, stirring until combined.

3. Heat coconut oil in a pan and cook pancakes until bubbles form, then flip and cook until golden brown.

Nutrition Information:
- Calories: 200
- Protein: 12g
- Carbohydrates: 30g
- Fat: 5g
- Fiber: 6g
- Sugar: 5g
- Portion Size: 2 pancakes

Lentil and Vegetable Breakfast Muffins

Ingredients:
- 1 cup cooked lentils
- 1/2 cup diced vegetables (bell peppers, spinach, onions)
- 2 eggs
- 1/4 cup grated cheese (optional)
- Salt and pepper to taste

Instructions:
1. Preheat oven to 350°F (175°C).

2. Mix cooked lentils, diced vegetables, eggs, cheese, salt, and pepper.

3. Spoon mixture into a greased muffin tin and bake for 20-25 minutes.

Nutrition Information:

- Calories: 150
- Protein: 10g
- Carbohydrates: 15g
- Fat: 6g
- Fiber: 5g
- Sugar: 2g
- Portion Size: 2 muffins

High-Protein Granola with Yogurt

Ingredients:

- 1/2 cup high-protein granola
- 1 cup Greek yogurt
- 1 tablespoon honey
- Fresh fruit for topping

Instructions:

1. Combine granola and Greek yogurt in a bowl.

2. Drizzle with honey and top with fresh fruit.

Nutrition Information:

- Calories: 300

- Protein: 20g

- Carbohydrates: 45g

- Fat: 8g

- Fiber: 5g

- Sugar: 25g

- Portion Size: 1 bowl

Edamame and Veggie Breakfast Wrap

Ingredients:

- 1 whole grain tortilla

- 1/2 cup shelled edamame

- 1/4 cup diced bell peppers

- 1/4 cup shredded carrots

- 2 tablespoons hummus

- Salt and pepper to taste

Instructions:

1. Spread hummus on the tortilla.

2. Add edamame, bell peppers, and carrots.

3. Season with salt and pepper, then roll up the wrap.

Nutrition Information:

- Calories: 250

- Protein: 12g

- Carbohydrates: 30g

- Fat: 8g

- Fiber: 8g

- Sugar: 4g

- Portion Size: 1 wrap

Baked Eggplant and Tomato Frittata

Ingredients:

- 1 small eggplant, diced

- 1/2 cup cherry tomatoes, halved

- 4 eggs

- 1/4 cup grated cheese

- 1 tablespoon olive oil

- Salt and pepper to taste

Instructions:

1. Preheat oven to 375°F (190°C).

2. Sauté eggplant in olive oil until tender, then transfer to a baking dish.

3. Add cherry tomatoes to the dish.

4. Beat eggs with cheese, salt, and pepper, then pour over vegetables.

5. Bake for 20-25 minutes.

Nutrition Information:

- Calories: 300
- Protein: 18g
- Carbohydrates: 12g
- Fat: 20g
- Fiber: 4g
- Sugar: 6g
- Portion Size: 2 slices

Almond Flour Breakfast Cookies

Ingredients:

- 1 cup almond flour
- 1/4 cup protein powder
- 1/4 cup almond butter
- 1/4 cup honey
- 1 teaspoon vanilla extract

- 1/2 teaspoon baking soda

Instructions:

1. Preheat oven to 350°F (175°C).
2. Mix all ingredients until combined.
3. Scoop dough onto a baking sheet and flatten slightly.
4. Bake for 10-12 minutes.

Nutrition Information:

- Calories: 150
- Protein: 8g
- Carbohydrates: 12g
- Fat: 10g
- Fiber: 3g
- Sugar: 8g
- Portion Size: 2 cookies

Chapter 3: Lunch Recipes

Lunch is an essential meal of the day, providing the energy and nutrients needed to power through the afternoon. For those managing Type 2 diabetes, a high-protein vegetarian lunch can help maintain blood sugar levels and keep hunger at bay. These recipes are designed to be nutritious, delicious, and easy to prepare.

Chickpea Salad with Lemon Tahini Dressing

Ingredients:

- 1 can chickpeas, rinsed and drained
- 1 cucumber, diced
- 1 cup cherry tomatoes, halved
- 1/4 red onion, finely chopped
- 1/4 cup parsley, chopped
- 2 tbsp tahini
- 1 lemon, juiced
- 1 clove garlic, minced
- Salt and pepper to taste

Instructions:

1. In a large bowl, combine chickpeas, cucumber, cherry tomatoes, red onion, and parsley.
2. In a small bowl, whisk together tahini, lemon juice, garlic, salt, and pepper.
3. Pour dressing over salad and toss to coat evenly.

Nutrition Information (per serving):

- Calories: 210
- Protein: 9g
- Carbohydrates: 30g
- Fat: 8g
- Fiber: 7g
- Sugar: 5g
- Portion Size: 1 cup

Grilled Portobello Mushroom Burger

Ingredients:

- 4 large portobello mushrooms
- 2 tbsp balsamic vinegar
- 2 tbsp olive oil
- 1 tsp dried oregano
- Salt and pepper to taste

- 4 whole grain burger buns
- Lettuce, tomato, and onion for topping

Instructions:

1. Preheat grill to medium-high heat.
2. In a small bowl, mix balsamic vinegar, olive oil, oregano, salt, and pepper.
3. Brush mushrooms with the marinade and let sit for 10 minutes.
4. Grill mushrooms for 5-7 minutes per side until tender.
5. Serve on buns with lettuce, tomato, and onion.

Nutrition Information (per serving):

- Calories: 250
- Protein: 7g
- Carbohydrates: 35g
- Fat: 10g
- Fiber: 5g
- Sugar: 6g
- Portion Size: 1 burger

Lentil and Sweet Potato Stew

Ingredients:

- 1 cup lentils, rinsed
- 2 sweet potatoes, peeled and cubed
- 1 onion, chopped
- 2 cloves garlic, minced
- 4 cups vegetable broth
- 1 tsp cumin
- 1 tsp paprika
- Salt and pepper to taste

Instructions:

1. In a large pot, sauté onion and garlic until softened.
2. Add lentils, sweet potatoes, vegetable broth, cumin, and paprika.
3. Bring to a boil, then reduce heat and simmer for 30 minutes.
4. Season with salt and pepper before serving.

Nutrition Information (per serving):

- Calories: 280
- Protein: 14g
- Carbohydrates: 50g
- Fat: 1g
- Fiber: 14g

- Sugar: 10g
- Portion Size: 1.5 cups

Quinoa and Black Bean Salad

Ingredients:

- 1 cup quinoa, cooked
- 1 can black beans, rinsed and drained
- 1 red bell pepper, diced
- 1/2 cup corn kernels
- 1/4 cup cilantro, chopped
- 2 tbsp olive oil
- 1 lime, juiced
- Salt and pepper to taste

Instructions:

1. In a large bowl, combine quinoa, black beans, bell pepper, corn, and cilantro.
2. In a small bowl, whisk together olive oil, lime juice, salt, and pepper.
3. Pour dressing over salad and toss to combine.

Nutrition Information (per serving):

- Calories: 290

- Protein: 10g

- Carbohydrates: 45g

- Fat: 10g

- Fiber: 9g

- Sugar: 4g

- Portion Size: 1.25 cups

Tofu and Vegetable Stir-Fry

Ingredients:

- 1 block firm tofu, cubed

- 2 tbsp soy sauce

- 1 tbsp sesame oil

- 2 cups mixed vegetables (bell peppers, broccoli, carrots)

- 2 cloves garlic, minced

- 1 tbsp ginger, minced

- 2 tbsp olive oil

Instructions:

1. In a bowl, marinate tofu in soy sauce for 10 minutes.

2. In a large pan, heat olive oil and sauté garlic and ginger until fragrant.

3. Add mixed vegetables and cook for 5-7 minutes.

4. Add tofu and cook for another 5 minutes, stirring frequently.

5. Drizzle with sesame oil before serving.

Nutrition Information (per serving):

- Calories: 220
- Protein: 14g
- Carbohydrates: 15g
- Fat: 14g
- Fiber: 5g
- Sugar: 5g
- Portion Size: 1.5 cups

Spinach and Chickpea Curry

Ingredients:

- 1 can chickpeas, rinsed and drained
- 2 cups fresh spinach
- 1 onion, chopped
- 2 cloves garlic, minced
- 1 can diced tomatoes
- 1 tbsp curry powder
- 1 cup coconut milk
- Salt and pepper to taste

Instructions:

1. In a large pot, sauté onion and garlic until softened.

2. Add chickpeas, diced tomatoes, curry powder, and coconut milk.

3. Simmer for 15 minutes.

4. Stir in spinach and cook until wilted.

5. Season with salt and pepper.

Nutrition Information (per serving):

- Calories: 240

- Protein: 8g

- Carbohydrates: 28g

- Fat: 12g

- Fiber: 8g

- Sugar: 7g

- Portion Size: 1.5 cups

Zucchini Noodles with Pesto and Edamame

Ingredients:

- 2 large zucchinis, spiralized

- 1 cup edamame, shelled

- 1/4 cup pesto sauce

- 1 tbsp olive oil

- Salt and pepper to taste

Instructions:

1. In a large pan, heat olive oil and sauté zucchini noodles for 2-3 minutes.

2. Add edamame and cook for another 2 minutes.

3. Stir in pesto sauce until noodles are coated.

4. Season with salt and pepper.

Nutrition Information (per serving):

- Calories: 200

- Protein: 10g

- Carbohydrates: 15g

- Fat: 14g

- Fiber: 4g

- Sugar: 5g

- Portion Size: 1.25 cups

Roasted Vegetable and Hummus Wrap

Ingredients:

- 1 red bell pepper, sliced

- 1 zucchini, sliced

- 1 red onion, sliced
- 1 tbsp olive oil
- Salt and pepper to taste
- 1 cup hummus
- 4 whole grain tortillas
- 1 cup spinach leaves

Instructions:

1. Preheat oven to 400°F (200°C).
2. Toss bell pepper, zucchini, and onion with olive oil, salt, and pepper.
3. Roast vegetables for 20 minutes until tender.
4. Spread hummus on tortillas, top with roasted vegetables and spinach.
5. Roll up and serve.

Nutrition Information (per serving):

- Calories: 280
- Protein: 8g
- Carbohydrates: 38g
- Fat: 12g
- Fiber: 8g
- Sugar: 6g
- Portion Size: 1 wrap

Cauliflower Rice and Bean Bowl

Ingredients:

- 1 head cauliflower, riced
- 1 can black beans, rinsed and drained
- 1 red bell pepper, diced
- 1 avocado, sliced
- 1 lime, juiced
- 1 tbsp olive oil
- Salt and pepper to taste

Instructions:

1. In a large pan, heat olive oil and sauté cauliflower rice for 5 minutes.
2. Add black beans and bell pepper, cook for another 5 minutes.
3. Drizzle with lime juice, season with salt and pepper.
4. Serve topped with avocado slices.

Nutrition Information (per serving):

- Calories: 250
- Protein: 9g
- Carbohydrates: 35g
- Fat: 10g
- Fiber: 11g
- Sugar: 5g

- Portion Size: 1.5 cups

Broccoli and Tempeh Salad

Ingredients:

- 1 block tempeh, cubed
- 2 cups broccoli florets
- 1/4 cup almonds, sliced
- 2 tbsp soy sauce
- 1 tbsp sesame oil
- 1 tbsp olive oil
- Salt and pepper to taste

Instructions:

1. In a bowl, marinate tempeh in soy sauce for 10 minutes.
2. In a large pan, heat olive oil and sauté tempeh until golden brown.
3. Steam broccoli until tender, about 5 minutes.
4. Combine tempeh, broccoli, and almonds in a bowl.
5. Drizzle with sesame oil, season with salt and pepper.

Nutrition Information (per serving):

- Calories: 300
- Protein: 18g

- Carbohydrates: 18g

- Fat: 18g

- Fiber: 7g

- Sugar: 3g

- Portion Size: 1.5 cups

Stuffed Bell Peppers with Quinoa and Beans

Ingredients:

- 4 bell peppers, tops cut off and seeds removed
- 1 cup cooked quinoa
- 1 can black beans, rinsed and drained
- 1 cup corn kernels
- 1/2 cup salsa
- 1 tsp cumin
- Salt and pepper to taste

Instructions:

1. Preheat oven to 375°F (190°C).
2. In a bowl, mix quinoa, black beans, corn, salsa, cumin, salt, and pepper.
3. Stuff bell peppers with the mixture.
4. Place in a baking dish and bake for 30 minutes.

Nutrition Information (per serving):

- Calories: 250
- Protein: 9g
- Carbohydrates: 45g
- Fat: 4g
- Fiber: 10g
- Sugar: 10g
- Portion Size: 1 pepper

Mushroom and Barley Soup

Ingredients:

- 1 cup barley
- 2 cups mushrooms, sliced
- 1 onion, chopped
- 2 cloves garlic, minced
- 4 cups vegetable broth
- 1 tbsp olive oil
- 1 tsp thyme
- Salt and pepper to taste

Instructions:

1. In a large pot, heat olive oil and sauté onion, garlic, and mushrooms until softened.

2. Add barley, vegetable broth, thyme, salt, and pepper.

3. Bring to a boil, then simmer for 40 minutes until barley is tender.

Nutrition Information (per serving):

- Calories: 220
- Protein: 6g
- Carbohydrates: 40g
- Fat: 5g
- Fiber: 8g
- Sugar: 6g
- Portion Size: 1.5 cups

Veggie Sushi Rolls with Tofu

Ingredients:

- 1 block firm tofu, sliced into strips
- 2 cups sushi rice, cooked
- 1 cucumber, julienned
- 1 carrot, julienned
- 1 avocado, sliced
- 4 sheets nori (seaweed)
- 2 tbsp soy sauce

Instructions:

1. Lay a sheet of nori on a bamboo mat.

2. Spread sushi rice evenly on nori, leaving a border.

3. Place tofu, cucumber, carrot, and avocado in the center.

4. Roll tightly, slice into pieces, and serve with soy sauce.

Nutrition Information (per serving):

- Calories: 300

- Protein: 10g

- Carbohydrates: 45g

- Fat: 8g

- Fiber: 6g

- Sugar: 4g

- Portion Size: 1 roll

Mediterranean Lentil Soup

Ingredients:

- 1 cup lentils, rinsed

- 1 can diced tomatoes

- 1 onion, chopped

- 2 cloves garlic, minced

- 4 cups vegetable broth

- 1 tsp oregano

- 1 tsp thyme

- Salt and pepper to taste

Instructions:

1. In a large pot, sauté onion and garlic until softened.

2. Add lentils, diced tomatoes, vegetable broth, oregano, and thyme.

3. Bring to a boil, then simmer for 30 minutes until lentils are tender.

4. Season with salt and pepper.

Nutrition Information (per serving):

- Calories: 250

- Protein: 12g

- Carbohydrates: 35g

- Fat: 4g

- Fiber: 10g

- Sugar: 8g

- Portion Size: 1.5 cups

Vegan Caesar Salad with Crispy Chickpeas

Ingredients:

- 1 can chickpeas, rinsed and drained
- 1 tbsp olive oil
- 1 tsp garlic powder
- 1 romaine lettuce, chopped
- 1/4 cup vegan Caesar dressing
- 1/4 cup nutritional yeast

Instructions:

1. Preheat oven to 400°F (200°C).
2. Toss chickpeas with olive oil and garlic powder.
3. Roast chickpeas for 20 minutes until crispy.
4. In a large bowl, combine lettuce, roasted chickpeas, and nutritional yeast.
5. Drizzle with Caesar dressing and toss to coat.

Nutrition Information (per serving):

- Calories: 220
- Protein: 8g
- Carbohydrates: 20g
- Fat: 12g
- Fiber: 6g

- Sugar: 4g
- Portion Size: 1.5 cups

Chapter 4: Dinner Recipes

When managing Type 2 diabetes, dinner is a crucial meal to focus on, ensuring it's balanced, satisfying, and supports blood sugar management. Here are fifteen high-protein, vegetarian dinner recipes that are not only nutritious but also delicious and easy to prepare.

Black Bean and Quinoa Tacos

Ingredients:

- 1 cup cooked quinoa
- 1 can black beans, drained and rinsed
- 1 tbsp olive oil
- 1 red bell pepper, diced
- 1 small onion, diced
- 2 cloves garlic, minced
- 1 tsp cumin
- 1 tsp chili powder
- Salt and pepper to taste
- Corn tortillas
- Fresh cilantro, chopped
- Lime wedges

Instructions:

1. Heat olive oil in a pan over medium heat. Add onion and garlic, sauté until softened.
2. Add bell pepper, cook for 5 minutes.
3. Stir in black beans, quinoa, cumin, chili powder, salt, and pepper. Cook until heated through.
4. Serve on corn tortillas, garnished with cilantro and lime wedges.

Nutrition Information:

- Calories: 200
- Protein: 8g
- Carbohydrates: 32g
- Fat: 5g
- Fiber: 8g
- Sugar: 2g
- Portion Size: 2 tacos

Eggplant Parmesan with Tofu

Ingredients:

- 1 large eggplant, sliced into rounds
- 1 block firm tofu, pressed and sliced
- 1 cup marinara sauce

- 1 cup vegan mozzarella cheese
- 1 cup whole wheat breadcrumbs
- 1 tsp Italian seasoning
- 2 tbsp olive oil
- Salt and pepper to taste

Instructions:

1. Preheat oven to 375°F (190°C).
2. Coat eggplant and tofu slices with olive oil, then with breadcrumbs mixed with Italian seasoning.
3. Place on a baking sheet and bake for 25 minutes until golden.
4. Layer eggplant, tofu, marinara sauce, and mozzarella in a baking dish.
5. Bake for an additional 20 minutes until cheese is melted and bubbly.

Nutrition Information:

- Calories: 300
- Protein: 15g
- Carbohydrates: 25g
- Fat: 15g
- Fiber: 6g
- Sugar: 6g
- Portion Size: 1 serving

Chickpea and Spinach Stew

Ingredients:

- 1 can chickpeas, drained and rinsed
- 4 cups fresh spinach
- 1 onion, chopped
- 2 cloves garlic, minced
- 1 can diced tomatoes
- 1 tsp cumin
- 1 tsp paprika
- 2 cups vegetable broth
- Salt and pepper to taste

Instructions:

1. Sauté onion and garlic in a pot until fragrant.
2. Add cumin and paprika, cook for 1 minute.
3. Stir in chickpeas, tomatoes, and vegetable broth. Simmer for 15 minutes.
4. Add spinach, cook until wilted. Season with salt and pepper.

Nutrition Information:

- Calories: 220
- Protein: 10g
- Carbohydrates: 35g
- Fat: 4g

- Fiber: 10g

- Sugar: 6g

- Portion Size: 1 bowl

Cauliflower Steaks with Lentil Sauce

Ingredients:

- 1 large cauliflower, cut into steaks

- 2 tbsp olive oil

- 1 cup cooked lentils

- 1 can diced tomatoes

- 1 onion, chopped

- 2 cloves garlic, minced

- 1 tsp cumin

- Salt and pepper to taste

Instructions:

1. Preheat oven to 400°F (200°C).

2. Brush cauliflower steaks with olive oil, season with salt and pepper. Roast for 20 minutes.

3. Sauté onion and garlic in a pan until softened.

4. Add cumin, lentils, and tomatoes. Simmer for 10 minutes.

5. Serve cauliflower steaks topped with lentil sauce.

Nutrition Information:

- Calories: 250
- Protein: 12g
- Carbohydrates: 35g
- Fat: 8g
- Fiber: 12g
- Sugar: 8g
- Portion Size: 1 steak

Vegan Shepherd's Pie with Lentils

Ingredients:

- 2 cups cooked lentils
- 1 onion, chopped
- 2 carrots, diced
- 1 cup peas
- 2 cups mashed potatoes
- 2 tbsp olive oil
- 1 tsp thyme
- Salt and pepper to taste

Instructions:

1. Preheat oven to 375°F (190°C).
2. Sauté onion and carrots in olive oil until tender.

3. Add lentils, peas, thyme, salt, and pepper. Cook for 5 minutes.

4. Transfer to a baking dish, top with mashed potatoes.

5. Bake for 25 minutes until golden.

Nutrition Information:

- Calories: 300
- Protein: 10g
- Carbohydrates: 50g
- Fat: 8g
- Fiber: 12g
- Sugar: 6g
- Portion Size: 1 slice

Stuffed Acorn Squash with Quinoa

Ingredients:

- 2 acorn squashes, halved and seeded
- 1 cup cooked quinoa
- 1 can black beans, drained and rinsed
- 1 red bell pepper, diced
- 1 onion, chopped
- 1 tsp cumin
- Salt and pepper to taste

- 2 tbsp olive oil

Instructions:

1. Preheat oven to 375°F (190°C).
2. Brush squash halves with olive oil, season with salt and pepper. Roast for 30 minutes.
3. Sauté onion and bell pepper in a pan until softened.
4. Add quinoa, black beans, cumin, salt, and pepper. Cook for 5 minutes.
5. Stuff squash halves with quinoa mixture. Bake for 10 minutes.

Nutrition Information:

- Calories: 350
- Protein: 10g
- Carbohydrates: 60g
- Fat: 10g
- Fiber: 15g
- Sugar: 6g
- Portion Size: 1 half squash

Tempeh and Vegetable Kebabs

Ingredients:

- 1 block tempeh, cubed
- 1 red bell pepper, cubed
- 1 zucchini, sliced
- 1 red onion, cubed
- 2 tbsp olive oil
- 1 tsp smoked paprika
- 1 tsp garlic powder
- Salt and pepper to taste

Instructions:

1. Preheat grill to medium-high heat.
2. Toss tempeh and vegetables with olive oil, smoked paprika, garlic powder, salt, and pepper.
3. Thread onto skewers.
4. Grill for 10 minutes, turning occasionally.

Nutrition Information:

- Calories: 250
- Protein: 15g
- Carbohydrates: 20g
- Fat: 12g
- Fiber: 6g

- Sugar: 5g
- Portion Size: 2 kebabs

Spaghetti Squash with Tomato and Basil

Ingredients:

- 1 spaghetti squash, halved and seeded
- 2 cups cherry tomatoes, halved
- 1/4 cup fresh basil, chopped
- 2 cloves garlic, minced
- 2 tbsp olive oil
- Salt and pepper to taste

Instructions:

1. Preheat oven to 375°F (190°C).
2. Brush squash with olive oil, season with salt and pepper. Roast for 40 minutes.
3. Sauté garlic in olive oil until fragrant.
4. Add tomatoes, cook until softened.
5. Scrape squash into strands, mix with tomato and basil mixture.

Nutrition Information:

- Calories: 180

- Protein: 4g

- Carbohydrates: 25g

- Fat: 8g

- Fiber: 6g

- Sugar: 8g

- Portion Size: 1 bowl

Mushroom Stroganoff with Tofu

Ingredients:

- 1 block firm tofu, cubed

- 2 cups mushrooms, sliced

- 1 onion, chopped

- 2 cloves garlic, minced

- 1 cup vegetable broth

- 1/2 cup unsweetened almond milk

- 2 tbsp olive oil

- 1 tbsp soy sauce

- 1 tsp thyme

- Salt and pepper to taste

Instructions:

1. Sauté onion, garlic, and mushrooms in olive oil until tender.

2. Add tofu, soy sauce, and thyme. Cook for 5 minutes.

3. Stir in vegetable broth and almond milk. Simmer for 10
   minutes.
4. Season with salt and pepper.

Nutrition Information:
- Calories: 220
- Protein: 12g
- Carbohydrates: 20g
- Fat: 10g
- Fiber: 4g
- Sugar: 3g
- Portion Size: 1 bowl

Lentil and Mushroom Bolognese

Ingredients:
- 1 cup lentils, cooked
- 2 cups mushrooms, chopped
- 1 onion, chopped
- 2 cloves garlic, minced
- 1 can crushed tomatoes
- 1 tbsp olive oil
- 1 tsp oregano
- Salt and pepper to taste

Instructions:

1. Sauté onion, garlic, and mushrooms in olive oil until tender.

2. Add lentils, tomatoes, and oregano. Simmer for 15 minutes.

3. Season with salt and pepper. Serve over whole grain pasta.

Nutrition Information:

- Calories: 200

- Protein: 10g

- Carbohydrates: 35g

- Fat: 5g

- Fiber: 8g

- Sugar: 6g

- Portion Size: 1 bowl

Vegan Moussaka with Eggplant and Lentils

Ingredients:

- 2 eggplants, sliced

- 1 cup lentils, cooked

- 1 onion, chopped

- 2 cloves garlic, minced

- 1 can diced tomatoes

- 1/2 cup vegan béchamel sauce

- 2 tbsp olive oil

- 1 tsp cinnamon

- Salt and pepper to taste

Instructions:

1. Preheat oven to 375°F (190°C).

2. Brush eggplant slices with olive oil, roast for 20 minutes.

3. Sauté onion and garlic until tender. Add lentils, tomatoes, cinnamon, salt, and pepper.

4. Layer eggplant and lentil mixture in a baking dish. Top with béchamel sauce.

5. Bake for 25 minutes until golden.

Nutrition Information:

- Calories: 300

- Protein: 12g

- Carbohydrates: 40g

- Fat: 12g

- Fiber: 10g

- Sugar: 8g

- Portion Size: 1 slice

Butternut Squash and Chickpea Curry

Ingredients:

- 1 butternut squash, peeled and cubed
- 1 can chickpeas, drained and rinsed
- 1 onion, chopped
- 2 cloves garlic, minced
- 1 can coconut milk
- 2 tbsp curry powder
- 1 tbsp olive oil
- Salt and pepper to taste

Instructions:

1. Sauté onion and garlic in olive oil until tender.
2. Add curry powder, cook for 1 minute.
3. Stir in butternut squash, chickpeas, and coconut milk. Simmer for 20 minutes until squash is tender.
4. Season with salt and pepper.

Nutrition Information:

- Calories: 350
- Protein: 10g
- Carbohydrates: 50g
- Fat: 15g
- Fiber: 10g

- Sugar: 10g

- Portion Size: 1 bowl

Vegan Pad Thai with Tofu

Ingredients:

- 1 block firm tofu, cubed

- 8 oz rice noodles

- 1 cup bean sprouts

- 1 red bell pepper, sliced

- 2 cloves garlic, minced

- 1/4 cup soy sauce

- 2 tbsp peanut butter

- 2 tbsp lime juice

- 1 tbsp olive oil

- 1 tbsp sriracha

- Fresh cilantro, chopped

Instructions:

1. Cook rice noodles according to package instructions.

2. Sauté garlic and tofu in olive oil until golden.

3. Add bell pepper, cook for 5 minutes.

4. Stir in soy sauce, peanut butter, lime juice, and sriracha. Cook until heated through.

5. Toss with noodles and bean sprouts. Garnish with cilantro.

Nutrition Information:

- Calories: 400
- Protein: 15g
- Carbohydrates: 50g
- Fat: 15g
- Fiber: 6g
- Sugar: 8g
- Portion Size: 1 bowl

Sweet Potato and Black Bean Enchiladas

Ingredients:

- 2 sweet potatoes, peeled and cubed
- 1 can black beans, drained and rinsed
- 1 onion, chopped
- 2 cloves garlic, minced
- 1 cup enchilada sauce
- 8 corn tortillas
- 1 cup vegan cheese
- 2 tbsp olive oil
- Salt and pepper to taste

Instructions:

1. Preheat oven to 375°F (190°C).

2. Sauté onion and garlic in olive oil until tender.

3. Add sweet potatoes, cook until softened. Stir in black beans.

4. Fill tortillas with sweet potato mixture, roll up and place in a baking dish.

5. Top with enchilada sauce and vegan cheese. Bake for 20 minutes.

Nutrition Information:

- Calories: 350

- Protein: 12g

- Carbohydrates: 50g

- Fat: 12g

- Fiber: 10g

- Sugar: 6g

- Portion Size: 2 enchiladas

Cauliflower and Chickpea Tikka Masala

Ingredients:

- 1 head cauliflower, cut into florets

- 1 can chickpeas, drained and rinsed

- 1 onion, chopped

- 2 cloves garlic, minced

- 1 can coconut milk

- 2 tbsp tikka masala paste

- 1 tbsp olive oil

- Salt and pepper to taste

Instructions:

1. Sauté onion and garlic in olive oil until tender.

2. Add tikka masala paste, cook for 1 minute.

3. Stir in cauliflower, chickpeas, and coconut milk. Simmer for 20 minutes until cauliflower is tender.

4. Season with salt and pepper.

Nutrition Information:

- Calories: 300

- Protein: 10g

- Carbohydrates: 35g

- Fat: 15g

- Fiber: 10g

- Sugar: 8g

- Portion Size: 1 bowl

Chapter 5: Snacks and Appetizers

Snacking can be a challenge for those with Type 2 diabetes, but it doesn't have to be. The key is to choose snacks that are high in protein, fiber, and healthy fats, while being low in simple carbohydrates. This chapter provides a variety of tasty, high-protein vegetarian snacks that will keep your blood sugar levels stable and your energy levels high.

Roasted Chickpeas

Ingredients:

- 1 can chickpeas, drained and rinsed
- 1 tbsp olive oil
- 1 tsp paprika
- 1 tsp garlic powder
- Salt and pepper to taste

Instructions:

1. Preheat oven to 400°F (200°C).
2. Toss chickpeas with olive oil, paprika, garlic powder, salt, and pepper.
3. Spread on a baking sheet and roast for 25-30 minutes, stirring occasionally, until crispy.

Nutrition Information (per serving):

- Calories: 120
- Protein: 5g
- Carbohydrates: 18g
- Fat: 3g
- Fiber: 5g
- Sugar: 1g
- Portion Size: 1/2 cup

Edamame Hummus with Veggies

Ingredients:

- 2 cups shelled edamame, cooked
- 1/4 cup tahini
- 1/4 cup lemon juice
- 2 garlic cloves
- 1/4 cup olive oil
- Salt to taste
- Assorted fresh veggies (carrots, cucumbers, bell peppers)

Instructions:

1. Blend edamame, tahini, lemon juice, and garlic in a food processor.
2. Slowly add olive oil until smooth.

3. Season with salt and serve with fresh veggies.

Nutrition Information (per serving):

- Calories: 150
- Protein: 8g
- Carbohydrates: 10g
- Fat: 9g
- Fiber: 4g
- Sugar: 2g
- Portion Size: 1/4 cup hummus with 1 cup veggies

Greek Yogurt with Cucumber and Dill

Ingredients:

- 1 cup Greek yogurt
- 1/2 cucumber, finely chopped
- 1 tbsp fresh dill, chopped
- 1 garlic clove, minced
- Salt and pepper to taste

Instructions:

1. Mix yogurt, cucumber, dill, and garlic in a bowl.
2. Season with salt and pepper.
3. Chill before serving.

Nutrition Information (per serving):

- Calories: 100
- Protein: 10g
- Carbohydrates: 5g
- Fat: 4g
- Fiber: 1g
- Sugar: 4g
- Portion Size: 1/2 cup

Spicy Tofu Bites

Ingredients:

- 1 block firm tofu, cubed
- 2 tbsp soy sauce
- 1 tbsp sriracha
- 1 tbsp olive oil
- 1 tsp garlic powder

Instructions:

1. Preheat oven to 375°F (190°C).
2. Toss tofu cubes with soy sauce, sriracha, olive oil, and garlic powder.
3. Spread on a baking sheet and bake for 20-25 minutes, until crispy.

Nutrition Information (per serving):

- Calories: 120
- Protein: 10g
- Carbohydrates: 4g
- Fat: 8g
- Fiber: 1g
- Sugar: 1g
- Portion Size: 1/2 cup

Almond and Seed Crackers

Ingredients:

- 1 cup almond flour
- 1/4 cup flaxseeds
- 1/4 cup chia seeds
- 1/2 tsp salt
- 1/4 cup water

Instructions:

1. Preheat oven to 350°F (175°C).
2. Mix all ingredients into a dough.
3. Roll out between two sheets of parchment paper.
4. Cut into squares and bake for 20 minutes, until golden.

Nutrition Information (per serving):

- Calories: 110
- Protein: 4g
- Carbohydrates: 6g
- Fat: 9g
- Fiber: 4g
- Sugar: 1g
- Portion Size: 4-5 crackers

Lentil and Vegetable Samosas

Ingredients:

- 1 cup cooked lentils
- 1 potato, diced and boiled
- 1/2 cup peas
- 1 onion, chopped
- 1 tbsp curry powder
- Phyllo dough sheets

Instructions:

1. Preheat oven to 375°F (190°C).
2. Mix lentils, potato, peas, onion, and curry powder.
3. Fill phyllo dough with mixture and fold into triangles.
4. Bake for 20-25 minutes, until crispy.

Nutrition Information (per serving):

- Calories: 140
- Protein: 5g
- Carbohydrates: 22g
- Fat: 3g
- Fiber: 4g
- Sugar: 2g
- Portion Size: 1 samosa

Stuffed Mini Peppers with Quinoa

Ingredients:

- 1 cup cooked quinoa
- 1/4 cup black beans
- 1/4 cup corn
- 12 mini bell peppers, halved and seeded
- 1/2 cup shredded cheese

Instructions:

1. Preheat oven to 375°F (190°C).
2. Mix quinoa, black beans, and corn.
3. Stuff mini peppers with the mixture.
4. Top with shredded cheese and bake for 15-20 minutes.

Nutrition Information (per serving):

- Calories: 130
- Protein: 5g
- Carbohydrates: 18g
- Fat: 5g
- Fiber: 4g
- Sugar: 3g
- Portion Size: 3 stuffed peppers

Baked Zucchini Chips

Ingredients:

- 2 zucchinis, thinly sliced
- 2 tbsp olive oil
- 1/4 cup grated Parmesan
- Salt and pepper to taste

Instructions:

1. Preheat oven to 250°F (120°C).
2. Toss zucchini slices with olive oil, Parmesan, salt, and pepper.
3. Arrange on a baking sheet and bake for 1.5-2 hours, until crispy.

Nutrition Information (per serving):

- Calories: 80
- Protein: 3g
- Carbohydrates: 4g
- Fat: 6g
- Fiber: 1g
- Sugar: 2g
- Portion Size: 1/2 cup

Guacamole with Veggie Sticks

Ingredients:

- 2 avocados, mashed
- 1/2 onion, chopped
- 1 tomato, chopped
- 1 lime, juiced
- Salt to taste
- Assorted veggie sticks (carrots, celery, bell peppers)

Instructions:

1. Mix avocados, onion, tomato, lime juice, and salt.
2. Serve with fresh veggie sticks.

Nutrition Information (per serving):

- Calories: 160
- Protein: 2g
- Carbohydrates: 12g
- Fat: 14g
- Fiber: 7g
- Sugar: 2g
- Portion Size: 1/4 cup guacamole with 1 cup veggies

Cottage Cheese and Herb Dip

Ingredients:

- 1 cup cottage cheese
- 1 tbsp fresh chives, chopped
- 1 tbsp fresh parsley, chopped
- 1 garlic clove, minced
- Salt and pepper to taste

Instructions:

1. Blend cottage cheese, chives, parsley, and garlic until smooth.
2. Season with salt and pepper and chill before serving.

Nutrition Information (per serving):

- Calories: 90
- Protein: 10g
- Carbohydrates: 3g
- Fat: 3g
- Fiber: 0g
- Sugar: 2g
- Portion Size: 1/2 cup

Spicy Black Bean Dip with Whole Grain Chips

Ingredients:

- 1 can black beans, drained and rinsed
- 1/4 cup salsa
- 1 tsp cumin
- 1 garlic clove, minced
- Whole grain chips

Instructions:

1. Blend black beans, salsa, cumin, and garlic until smooth.
2. Serve with whole grain chips.

Nutrition Information (per serving):

- Calories: 150
- Protein: 6g
- Carbohydrates: 20g
- Fat: 5g
- Fiber: 6g
- Sugar: 1g
- Portion Size: 1/4 cup dip with 1 ounce chips

Kale and Chickpea Chips

Ingredients:

- 1 bunch kale, torn into pieces
- 1 can chickpeas, drained and rinsed
- 2 tbsp olive oil
- 1 tsp paprika
- Salt to taste

Instructions:

1. Preheat oven to 375°F (190°C).
2. Toss kale and chickpeas with olive oil, paprika, and salt.
3. Spread on a baking sheet and bake for 15-20 minutes, until crispy.

Nutrition Information (per serving):

- Calories: 110
- Protein: 4g
- Carbohydrates: 14g
- Fat: 5g
- Fiber: 4g
- Sugar: 1g
- Portion Size: 1/2 cup

Veggie and Tofu Skewers

Ingredients:

- 1 block firm tofu, cubed
- 1 zucchini, sliced
- 1 bell pepper, chopped
- 1 red onion, chopped
- 2 tbsp olive oil
- 1 tbsp soy sauce

Instructions:

1. Preheat grill to medium-high heat.
2. Thread tofu, zucchini, bell pepper, and onion onto skewers.
3. Brush with olive oil and soy sauce.
4. Grill for 10-15 minutes, turning occasionally.

Nutrition Information (per serving):

- Calories: 120
- Protein: 8g
- Carbohydrates: 6g
- Fat: 8g
- Fiber: 2g
- Sugar: 3g
- Portion Size: 2 skewers

Almond Butter and Banana Bites

Ingredients:

- 2 bananas, sliced
- 1/4 cup almond butter

Instructions:

1. Spread almond butter on banana slices.
2. Sandwich slices together.

Nutrition Information (per serving):

- Calories: 150
- Protein: 4g
- Carbohydrates: 22g
- Fat: 7g

- Fiber: 3g

- Sugar: 12g

- Portion Size: 6 bites

Protein-Packed Energy Balls

Ingredients:

- 1 cup oats

- 1/2 cup peanut butter

- 1/4 cup honey

- 1/4 cup protein powder

- 1/4 cup dark chocolate chips

Instructions:

1. Mix all ingredients in a bowl.

2. Roll into balls and chill before serving.

Nutrition Information (per serving):

- Calories: 100

- Protein: 5g

- Carbohydrates: 12g

- Fat: 5g

- Fiber: 2g

- Sugar: 6g

- Portion Size: 2 balls

Chapter 6: Desserts

Desserts don't have to be guilty pleasures; they can be nutritious and delicious at the same time. The following recipes are crafted to satisfy your sweet tooth while providing wholesome ingredients and balanced nutrition. Each dessert is designed to be simple yet delightful, perfect for any occasion.

Chia Seed Pudding with Cocoa

Ingredients:

- 1/4 cup chia seeds
- 1 cup almond milk
- 2 tbsp cocoa powder
- 1 tbsp maple syrup
- 1 tsp vanilla extract

Instructions:

1. Mix all ingredients in a bowl.
2. Stir well to combine.
3. Refrigerate for at least 4 hours or overnight.

Nutrition Information:

- Calories: 180

- Protein: 5g

- Carbohydrates: 18g

- Fat: 10g

- Fiber: 12g

- Sugar: 6g

- Portion Size: 1 serving

Almond Flour Brownies

Ingredients:

- 1 cup almond flour

- 1/2 cup cocoa powder

- 1/2 cup coconut sugar

- 1/4 cup melted coconut oil

- 2 eggs

- 1 tsp vanilla extract

Instructions:

1. Preheat oven to 350°F (175°C).

2. Combine all ingredients in a bowl.

3. Pour mixture into a baking dish.

4. Bake for 20-25 minutes.

Nutrition Information:

- Calories: 210
- Protein: 6g
- Carbohydrates: 18g
- Fat: 15g
- Fiber: 4g
- Sugar: 10g
- Portion Size: 1 brownie

Vegan Protein Cookies

Ingredients:

- 1 cup oat flour
- 1/2 cup protein powder
- 1/4 cup almond butter
- 1/4 cup maple syrup
- 1/4 cup almond milk
- 1 tsp baking powder
- 1 tsp vanilla extract

Instructions:

1. Preheat oven to 350°F (175°C).
2. Mix all ingredients in a bowl.
3. Scoop dough onto a baking sheet.

4. Bake for 12-15 minutes.

Nutrition Information:

- Calories: 150
- Protein: 8g
- Carbohydrates: 18g
- Fat: 6g
- Fiber: 3g
- Sugar: 6g
- Portion Size: 1 cookie

Greek Yogurt with Honey and Walnuts

Ingredients:

- 1 cup Greek yogurt
- 1 tbsp honey
- 2 tbsp chopped walnuts

Instructions:

1. Scoop yogurt into a bowl.
2. Drizzle with honey.
3. Sprinkle with walnuts.

Nutrition Information:

- Calories: 200
- Protein: 15g
- Carbohydrates: 18g
- Fat: 8g
- Fiber: 1g
- Sugar: 14g
- Portion Size: 1 serving

Black Bean Brownies

Ingredients:

- 1 can black beans (rinsed and drained)
- 2 eggs
- 1/2 cup cocoa powder
- 1/2 cup coconut sugar
- 1/4 cup coconut oil
- 1 tsp vanilla extract

Instructions:

1. Preheat oven to 350°F (175°C).
2. Blend all ingredients until smooth.
3. Pour into a baking dish.
4. Bake for 20-25 minutes.

Nutrition Information:

- Calories: 190
- Protein: 5g
- Carbohydrates: 26g
- Fat: 8g
- Fiber: 5g
- Sugar: 14g
- Portion Size: 1 brownie

Tofu Chocolate Mousse

Ingredients:

- 1 block silken tofu
- 1/2 cup melted dark chocolate
- 2 tbsp maple syrup
- 1 tsp vanilla extract

Instructions:

1. Blend all ingredients until smooth.
2. Chill for 1 hour before serving.

Nutrition Information:

- Calories: 160
- Protein: 7g

- Carbohydrates: 18g
- Fat: 8g
- Fiber: 2g
- Sugar: 12g
- Portion Size: 1 serving

Peanut Butter Protein Balls

Ingredients:

- 1 cup rolled oats
- 1/2 cup peanut butter
- 1/4 cup honey
- 1/4 cup protein powder
- 1 tsp vanilla extract

Instructions:

1. Mix all ingredients in a bowl.
2. Roll into balls.
3. Chill for 1 hour before serving.

Nutrition Information:

- Calories: 100
- Protein: 5g
- Carbohydrates: 12g

- Fat: 4g

- Fiber: 2g

- Sugar: 7g

- Portion Size: 1 ball

Avocado Chocolate Pudding

Ingredients:

- 2 ripe avocados

- 1/4 cup cocoa powder

- 1/4 cup maple syrup

- 1 tsp vanilla extract

Instructions:

1. Blend all ingredients until smooth.

2. Chill for 1 hour before serving.

Nutrition Information:

- Calories: 200

- Protein: 3g

- Carbohydrates: 28g

- Fat: 12g

- Fiber: 9g

- Sugar: 15g

- Portion Size: 1 serving

Baked Apple with Cinnamon and Nuts

Ingredients:

- 2 apples, cored
- 2 tbsp chopped nuts
- 1 tbsp maple syrup
- 1 tsp cinnamon

Instructions:

1. Preheat oven to 350°F (175°C).
2. Stuff apples with nuts.
3. Drizzle with maple syrup and sprinkle with cinnamon.
4. Bake for 20-25 minutes.

Nutrition Information:

- Calories: 150
- Protein: 2g
- Carbohydrates: 26g
- Fat: 6g
- Fiber: 5g
- Sugar: 18g
- Portion Size: 1 apple

Vegan Protein Cheesecake

Ingredients:

- 1 cup cashews, soaked
- 1/2 cup coconut cream
- 1/4 cup maple syrup
- 1/4 cup lemon juice
- 1/4 cup protein powder
- 1 tsp vanilla extract

Instructions:

1. Blend all ingredients until smooth.
2. Pour into a crust of choice.
3. Chill for at least 4 hours.

Nutrition Information:

- Calories: 250
- Protein: 8g
- Carbohydrates: 22g
- Fat: 15g
- Fiber: 2g
- Sugar: 14g
- Portion Size: 1 slice

Chocolate-Covered Almonds

Ingredients:

- 1 cup almonds
- 1/2 cup dark chocolate chips
- 1 tsp sea salt

Instructions:

1. Melt chocolate chips.
2. Dip almonds in melted chocolate.
3. Sprinkle with sea salt.
4. Chill until set.

Nutrition Information:

- Calories: 200
- Protein: 5g
- Carbohydrates: 15g
- Fat: 14g
- Fiber: 4g
- Sugar: 8g
- Portion Size: 1/4 cup

Coconut and Almond Macaroons

Ingredients:

- 2 cups shredded coconut
- 1 cup almond flour
- 1/2 cup maple syrup
- 1 tsp vanilla extract

Instructions:

1. Preheat oven to 325°F (160°C).
2. Mix all ingredients in a bowl.
3. Scoop onto a baking sheet.
4. Bake for 15-20 minutes.

Nutrition Information:

- Calories: 120
- Protein: 2g
- Carbohydrates: 12g
- Fat: 8g
- Fiber: 3g
- Sugar: 8g
- Portion Size: 1 macaroon

Protein-Packed Banana Bread

Ingredients:

- 2 ripe bananas
- 1 cup oat flour
- 1/2 cup protein powder
- 1/4 cup almond milk
- 1/4 cup maple syrup
- 1 tsp baking soda
- 1 tsp vanilla extract

Instructions:

1. Preheat oven to 350°F (175°C).
2. Mash bananas and mix with all other ingredients.
3. Pour into a loaf pan.
4. Bake for 30-35 minutes.

Nutrition Information:

- Calories: 180
- Protein: 7g
- Carbohydrates: 28g
- Fat: 4g
- Fiber: 4g
- Sugar: 12g
- Portion Size: 1 slice

Carrot Cake Bites

Ingredients:

- 1 cup grated carrots
- 1 cup oat flour
- 1/2 cup dates, pitted
- 1/4 cup almond butter
- 1 tsp cinnamon

Instructions:

1. Blend all ingredients until combined.
2. Roll into balls.
3. Chill for 1 hour before serving.

Nutrition Information:

- Calories: 100
- Protein: 2g
- Carbohydrates: 18g
- Fat: 3g
- Fiber: 3g
- Sugar: 12g
- Portion Size: 1 ball

High-Protein Berry Crumble

Ingredients:

- 2 cups mixed berries
- 1/2 cup rolled oats
- 1/4 cup almond flour
- 1/4 cup protein powder
- 1/4 cup maple syrup
- 2 tbsp coconut oil, melted

Instructions:

1. Preheat oven to 350°F (175°C).
2. Mix berries and maple syrup, place in a baking dish.
3. Combine oats, almond flour, protein powder, and coconut oil, sprinkle over berries.
4. Bake for 25-30 minutes.

Nutrition Information:

- Calories: 150
- Protein: 6g
- Carbohydrates: 24g
- Fat: 5g
- Fiber: 4g
- Sugar: 12g
- Portion Size: 1 serving

Chapter 7: Smoothies

Smoothies are an excellent way to pack a variety of nutrients into a single meal or snack. They can be tailored to suit your taste preferences and dietary needs, making them a versatile addition to any diet. In this chapter, we'll explore unique smoothie recipes that not only taste great but also provide a range of health benefits.

Spinach and Avocado Smoothie

Ingredients:

- 1 cup fresh spinach
- 1/2 ripe avocado
- 1 banana
- 1 cup unsweetened almond milk
- 1 tablespoon honey
- 1/2 cup ice

Instructions:

1. Combine all ingredients in a blender.
2. Blend until smooth.
3. Serve immediately.

Nutrition Information (per serving):

- Calories: 210
- Protein: 3g
- Carbohydrates: 32g
- Fat: 9g
- Fiber: 7g
- Sugar: 18g
- Portion size: 1 large smoothie

Berry and Chia Seed Smoothie

Ingredients:

- 1 cup mixed berries (strawberries, blueberries, raspberries)
- 1 tablespoon chia seeds
- 1 cup coconut water
- 1 tablespoon honey
- 1/2 cup ice

Instructions:

1. Add all ingredients to a blender.
2. Blend until smooth.
3. Enjoy immediately.

Nutrition Information (per serving):

- Calories: 160
- Protein: 2g
- Carbohydrates: 36g
- Fat: 2g
- Fiber: 8g
- Sugar: 24g
- Portion size: 1 large smoothie

Green Protein Smoothie

Ingredients:

- 1 cup kale leaves
- 1 scoop vanilla protein powder
- 1 banana
- 1 cup unsweetened almond milk
- 1 tablespoon flaxseed meal
- 1/2 cup ice

Instructions:

1. Blend all ingredients together until smooth.
2. Serve immediately.

Nutrition Information (per serving):

- Calories: 250
- Protein: 20g
- Carbohydrates: 30g
- Fat: 6g
- Fiber: 6g
- Sugar: 15g
- Portion size: 1 large smoothie

Peanut Butter and Banana Smoothie

Ingredients:

- 1 banana
- 1 tablespoon peanut butter
- 1 cup unsweetened almond milk
- 1 tablespoon honey
- 1/2 cup ice

Instructions:

1. Combine all ingredients in a blender.
2. Blend until smooth.
3. Serve immediately.

Nutrition Information (per serving):

- Calories: 250
- Protein: 5g
- Carbohydrates: 37g
- Fat: 10g
- Fiber: 4g
- Sugar: 24g
- Portion size: 1 large smoothie

Mango and Coconut Protein Smoothie

Ingredients:

- 1 cup frozen mango chunks
- 1 scoop vanilla protein powder
- 1 cup coconut milk
- 1 tablespoon chia seeds
- 1/2 cup ice

Instructions:

1. Add all ingredients to a blender.
2. Blend until smooth.
3. Enjoy immediately.

Nutrition Information (per serving):

- Calories: 300
- Protein: 18g
- Carbohydrates: 42g
- Fat: 10g
- Fiber: 6g
- Sugar: 30g
- Portion size: 1 large smoothie

Chocolate and Almond Smoothie

Ingredients:

- 1 scoop chocolate protein powder
- 1 tablespoon almond butter
- 1 banana
- 1 cup unsweetened almond milk
- 1/2 cup ice

Instructions:

1. Blend all ingredients until smooth.
2. Serve immediately.

Nutrition Information (per serving):

- Calories: 280

- Protein: 20g

- Carbohydrates: 30g

- Fat: 12g

- Fiber: 5g

- Sugar: 15g

- Portion size: 1 large smoothie

Blueberry and Flaxseed Smoothie

Ingredients:

- 1 cup blueberries

- 1 tablespoon ground flaxseed

- 1 cup unsweetened almond milk

- 1 tablespoon honey

- 1/2 cup ice

Instructions:

1. Combine all ingredients in a blender.

2. Blend until smooth.

3. Serve immediately.

Nutrition Information (per serving):

- Calories: 180

- Protein: 3g

- Carbohydrates: 36g

- Fat: 4g

- Fiber: 7g

- Sugar: 22g

- Portion size: 1 large smoothie

Strawberry and Tofu Smoothie

Ingredients:

- 1 cup strawberries

- 1/2 cup silken tofu

- 1 banana

- 1 cup unsweetened almond milk

- 1/2 cup ice

Instructions:

1. Blend all ingredients together until smooth.

2. Serve immediately.

Nutrition Information (per serving):

- Calories: 200

- Protein: 8g

- Carbohydrates: 35g

- Fat: 5g

- Fiber: 5g

- Sugar: 20g

- Portion size: 1 large smoothie

Kale and Pineapple Smoothie

Ingredients:

- 1 cup kale leaves

- 1 cup pineapple chunks

- 1 banana

- 1 cup coconut water

- 1/2 cup ice

Instructions:

1. Add all ingredients to a blender.

2. Blend until smooth.

3. Enjoy immediately.

Nutrition Information (per serving):

- Calories: 180

- Protein: 3g

- Carbohydrates: 42g

- Fat: 1g

- Fiber: 7g

- Sugar: 28g
- Portion size: 1 large smoothie

Apple and Cinnamon Protein Smoothie

Ingredients:

- 1 apple, cored and chopped
- 1 scoop vanilla protein powder
- 1/2 teaspoon cinnamon
- 1 cup unsweetened almond milk
- 1/2 cup ice

Instructions:

1. Combine all ingredients in a blender.
2. Blend until smooth.
3. Serve immediately.

Nutrition Information (per serving):

- Calories: 220
- Protein: 20g
- Carbohydrates: 30g
- Fat: 4g
- Fiber: 5g
- Sugar: 20g

- Portion size: 1 large smoothie

Mixed Berry and Greek Yogurt Smoothie

Ingredients:

- 1 cup mixed berries (strawberries, blueberries, raspberries)
- 1/2 cup Greek yogurt
- 1 cup unsweetened almond milk
- 1 tablespoon honey
- 1/2 cup ice

Instructions:

1. Blend all ingredients together until smooth.
2. Serve immediately.

Nutrition Information (per serving):

- Calories: 220
- Protein: 10g
- Carbohydrates: 36g
- Fat: 4g
- Fiber: 6g
- Sugar: 26g
- Portion size: 1 large smoothie

Orange and Carrot Protein Smoothie

Ingredients:

- 1 orange, peeled and segmented
- 1/2 cup grated carrots
- 1 scoop vanilla protein powder
- 1 cup coconut water
- 1/2 cup ice

Instructions:

1. Combine all ingredients in a blender.
2. Blend until smooth.
3. Serve immediately.

Nutrition Information (per serving):

- Calories: 200
- Protein: 20g
- Carbohydrates: 30g
- Fat: 2g
- Fiber: 6g
- Sugar: 22g
- Portion size: 1 large smoothie

Beetroot and Berry Smoothie

Ingredients:

- 1 small beetroot, peeled and chopped
- 1 cup mixed berries (strawberries, blueberries, raspberries)
- 1 banana
- 1 cup coconut water
- 1/2 cup ice

Instructions:

1. Add all ingredients to a blender.
2. Blend until smooth.
3. Enjoy immediately.

Nutrition Information (per serving):

- Calories: 170
- Protein: 3g
- Carbohydrates: 40g
- Fat: 1g
- Fiber: 7g
- Sugar: 28g
- Portion size: 1 large smoothie

Oatmeal and Cinnamon Smoothie

Ingredients:

- 1/2 cup rolled oats
- 1 banana
- 1/2 teaspoon cinnamon
- 1 cup unsweetened almond milk
- 1 tablespoon honey
- 1/2 cup ice

Instructions:

1. Combine all ingredients in a blender.
2. Blend until smooth.
3. Serve immediately.

Nutrition Information (per serving):

- Calories: 250
- Protein: 5g
- Carbohydrates: 50g
- Fat: 5g
- Fiber: 7g
- Sugar: 22g
- Portion size: 1 large smoothie

Pumpkin Spice Protein Smoothie

Ingredients:

- 1/2 cup pumpkin puree
- 1 scoop vanilla protein powder
- 1/2 teaspoon pumpkin pie spice
- 1 cup unsweetened almond milk
- 1 tablespoon honey
- 1/2 cup ice

Instructions:

1. Add all ingredients to a blender.
2. Blend until smooth.
3. Enjoy immediately.

Nutrition Information (per serving):

- Calories: 220
- Protein: 20g
- Carbohydrates: 30g
- Fat: 4g
- Fiber: 5g
- Sugar: 20g
- Portion size: 1 large smoothie

CONCLUSION

Congratulations on completing "Vegetarian High Protein Recipes for Type 2 Diabetics"! This book was crafted with the aim of providing you with not just recipes, but a comprehensive guide to managing your diabetes through delicious and nutritious vegetarian meals. As you've discovered throughout these pages, a high-protein diet can play a crucial role in stabilizing blood sugar levels and promoting overall health.

In this journey, you've explored a diverse range of recipes meticulously designed to be both satisfying and diabetes-friendly. From hearty breakfasts to wholesome dinners, from energizing smoothies to guilt-free desserts and snacks, each dish was chosen not only for its taste but also for its nutritional benefits.

Remember, managing diabetes is not just about what you eat, but how you approach your lifestyle. By incorporating these recipes into your daily routine, you've taken a proactive step towards better health. Planning your meals, experimenting with new ingredients, and enjoying the process of cooking can all contribute to your well-being.

As you move forward, continue to listen to your body and monitor how different foods affect your glucose levels. Stay connected with healthcare professionals for personalized guidance and support. Building a sustainable diet that works for you is key, and this book is here to serve as a foundation for your journey.

Lastly, stay inspired! Embrace the creativity and variety in vegetarian cooking. Whether you're preparing a quick snack or a special dinner, let each meal be an opportunity to nourish yourself and celebrate the flavors of wholesome ingredients.

Thank you for choosing "Vegetarian High Protein Recipes for Type 2 Diabetics". Here's to your health, happiness, and delicious meals ahead!